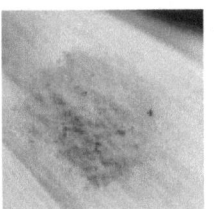

Table of contents:

Imprint:

Summary:

The spice turmeric plays an important role in the culinary world as well as in science and medicine. It has been shown that turmeric may have positive effects in the treatment of metabolic syndrome, inflammatory diseases such as arthritis, as well as hyperlipidaemia (increased blood lipids). Likewise, this plant is credited with possibly improving the performance of active people. Although it has been shown in scientific studies that the intake of curcumin alone, due to low absorption or a rapid metabolism and rapid elimination does not lead to the associated health benefits, ingredients such as the carrier of black pepper flavor lead to an improved bioavailability. Not least beneficial effects in terms of tumorigenesis (carcinogenesis) and inflammatory diseases such as psoriasis in the mouse model are assumed.

However, those study results that show possible effects of turmeric in animal experiments are not automatically transferable to humans. Opposing scientific work has also shown potential negative effects of turmeric on tumor growth in a medical context. The data available with regard to a benefit / risk assessment of turmeric seems therefore currently not clear. The aim of this book is to give an overview of the effects of turmeric on the human body, with references to current scientific literature. (1-3, 39)

Introduction:

Turmeric is a spice from the ginger family and has been known to man for several thousand years. The plant has significance in the culinary world as well as in science and medicine. Curcuma longa is traditionally used as a medicinal plant in Asian countries for its potential anti-inflammatory, antioxidant, antimutagenic, antimicrobial and anti-cancer properties. (4-11) Curcumin (plant yellow dye) is used as a dye for therapeutic purposes as well as a food. (12) The intake of curcumin and its potential health benefits seem to be primarily due to anti-inflammatory and antioxidant effects. (5)

Curcumin is a polyphenol that interacts with various signal molecules and also exhibits activity at the cellular level. (5) Potentially positive effects could be demonstrated with regard to metabolic syndrome, inflammatory diseases, pain, as well as eye diseases. (6-10) Although many beneficial effects of curcumin supplementation have been shown, one of the major problems with the use of curcumin itself is its poor bioavailability. This is caused by rapid metabolism, poor absorption and rapid elimination. As a result, various substances have been tested, which should increase the bioavailability of curcumin, i.a. the substance piperine (main ingredient of black pepper), which has an effect in this context. The addition of piperine (formation of a curcumin complex) thus allows the bioavailability of curcumin to be correspondingly improved. (5, 6, 13-15)

Curcumin is used in a variety of applications, such as curries in India, cosmetics in Thailand, or tea in Japan. In Malaysia it is used as an antiseptic, in China it is used as a dye. In the US, the spice is used in the food industry as a preservative and dye. (5) Curcumin is available in various forms, including tablets, ointments, energy drinks, etc., [5]

Mechanisms of action:

Potential antioxidative and anti-inflammatory properties of curcumin:

Possible antioxidant and antiinflammatory effects are major components of the mechanisms of action of curcumin. (16, 17) Evidence has been found in scientific studies that antioxidant components, e.g. the so-called superoxide dismutase can be increased by curcumin. (18-20) Furthermore, curcumin is able to influence free radicals and to inhibit or modulate related enzymes. (16, 17, 19)

Oxidative   stress:
Oxidative stress is an important component of many chronic diseases and is closely associated with inflammation. (21) In addition, a series of reactive oxygen / nitrogen species can trigger an intracellular signaling cascade that promotes proinflammatory gene expression. Diseases associated therewith are e.g. multiple sclerosis (MS), Alzheimer's disease, colitis, arthritis, cardiovascular disease, etc .. (20, 22-24) An important factor that plays a role in inflammatory activity is (NF) -κB (this inflammatory factor is activated by, for example, Gram-negative bacteria, various pathogenic viruses, UV radiation, cigarette smoking, including disease-causing factors). It has been shown that curcumin blocks the activation of NF-κB. It has also been shown that curcumin suppresses inflammation by many different mechanisms, supporting its mechanism of action as a potential anti-inflammatory agent. (20) Study results also suggest that curcumin supplementation significantly reduces serum concentrations of proinflammatory cytokines in patients with metabolic syndrome. (20)

Arthritis:

With regard to arthritis (painful inflammatory joint disease) it has been shown that after 8-12 weeks of standardized turmeric extract intake (typically 1000 mg / day curcumin), symptoms (mainly pain and inflammation-related symptoms) could be reduced. Therefore, turmeric extracts and curcumin may be recommended to relieve symptoms of arthritis, especially osteoarthritis. (25) Extensive research in the last half-century has provided important insights into curcumin.

Curcumin binds to a variety of proteins and inhibits the activity of various kinases. By modulating the activation of various transcription factors, curcumin also regulates the expression of inflammatory enzymes, cytokines, adhesion molecules and cell survival proteins. (26)

Neuroprotection:

Experimental data has highlighted the pleiotropic neuroprotective effects of curcumin due to its activity in several antioxidant and antiinflammatory pathways involved in neurodegeneration.

Although the poor systemic bioavailability of curcumin following oral administration and low plasma concentrations are limiting factors in therapeutic efficacy, innovative delivery formulations have been developed to overcome these limitations. (29)

It is believed that depression is a neuropsychiatric disorder, which may also include neuroinflammation in certain brain regions. (30)

Curcumin has potential neuroprotective properties and has shown a possible antidepressant-like effect in various animal models related to depression. (31-33) However, underlying mechanisms, in particular whether curcumin exerts neuroprotection by suppressing the activity of the inflammatory pathway in depression, are largely unknown.

In a recent study (34) it was shown that the repeated administration of curcumin (40 mg / kg, ip, 5 weeks) significantly increased the expression of the pro-inflammatory cytokine interleukin-1β (IL-1β) and the inhibition of neuronal apoptosis within neurons decreased (in the entromedial prefrontal cortex (vmPFC)). Depression-like behavior was improved.

In summary, these results indicate that curcumin may protect against IL-1β-induced neuronal apoptosis, which may be related to the occurrence of depression-like behaviors in stressed rats. In addition, they provide new insights into the mechanisms and therapeutic potential of curcumin in the treatment of inflammatory neuronal deterioration of this disease. (34)

Effects of curcumin on tumors:

Curcumin has been shown to have potential protective effects in several human cancers, including prostate, head and neck, melanoma, breast, colon and pancreatic cancer. [6] This concerns the inhibition of cancer growth and metastasis including other factors. [16, 42, 43]

Epidemiological studies have shown that the low incidence of colorectal cancer in India may be due to the chemopreventive and antioxidant properties of curcumin. [44]

The underlying mechanisms are comprehensive and diverse.

In addition, study results suggest (35) that curcumin may inhibit VEGF expression (vascular endothelial growth factor, which plays an important role in angiogenesis or tumor growth). (35) Study results also point to a possible anti-migration or anti-invasion effect of tumor cells by curcumin in the animal model. (37)

Study evidence supports the hypothesis that curcumin may inhibit memory and behavioral changes associated with ethanol poisoning. (36) Curcumin may therefore serve as a potential, promising, and cheap available neuroprotective compound against ethanol-associated neurodegenerative diseases. (36)

Effects of curcumin on sugar metabolism:

Study results showed that curcumin in combination with metformin (anti-diabetes drug) could act synergistically on dyslipidemia (disturbed lipid metabolism) and oxidative stress. Therefore, curcumin is a potentially promising strategy for the treatment of diabetic complications, mainly in the context of cardiovascular events. (38)

Side effects of curcumin:

There ia long experience with the use of curcumin. For example, the daily allowable intake of curcumin is between 0 and 3 mg / kg body weight, according to reports by JECFA (the United Nations Food and Feed Organization and the World Health Organization) and EFSA (European Food Safety Authority). (27)

Several studies in healthy volunteers have described the safety and efficacy of curcumin. Despite this generally accepted safety, some undesirable effects have been reported. These include diarrhea, headache, rash and yellow stools (22), as well as nausea and an increase in the levels of alkaline phosphatase and lactate dehydrogenase in the serum. (28)

Potential negative effects of curcumin in a medical context:

Many of the study results cited in this book were evident in animal experiments. However, the described effects of turmeric in a medical context are not automatically transferable to humans and should be interpreted with caution. Scientific papers have also shown adverse effects of turmeric in terms of tumor growth. (39)

Thus, on the one hand, potential protective properties of turmeric with regard to medicinal effects were demonstrated, as well as potentially negative results.

The data on a benefit / risk assessment of turmeric in connection with medical use seems therefore currently not clear and further research seems to be required in this regard.

Conclusion:

Due to its potential antioxidant and anti-inflammatory properties, curcumin has attracted worldwide attention.

These potential benefits are best achieved by combining curcumin with drugs such as piperine, which significantly increases bioavailability. Studies suggest that curcumin may be useful in the treatment of oxidative and inflammatory diseases, metabolic syndrome, arthritis, and hyperlipidemia, among others. (1, 34-38) However, many of the currently available scientific papers are reproducible only in animal experiments and it is therefore questionable whether these results are directly transferable to humans.

In addition, negative effects of curcumin have also been demonstrated (among other things regarding tumor behavior), which currently does not clarify a final benefit / risk profile of curcumin in a medical context.

Further studies therefore seem essential.

References:

1. Hewlings SJ, Kalman DS. Curcumin: A Review of Its' Effects on Human Health.Foods. 2017 Oct 22;6(10). pii: E92.

2. Ramirez-Boscá A, Soler A et al. Antioxidant Curcuma extracts decrease the blood lipid peroxide

levels of human subjects. AGE. 1995; 18 (4). pp 167–169|

3. Miquel J, Bernd A, Sempere JM, Díaz-Alperi J, Ramírez A. The curcuma antioxidants: pharm acological effects and prospects fo r future clinical use. A review. Arch Gerontol Geriatr. 2002 Feb;34(1):37-46.

4. Priyadarsini K.I. The chemistry of curcumin: From extraction to therapeutic
agent. Molecules. 2014;19:20091 –20112

5. Gupta S.C., Patchva S., Aggarwal B.B. Therapeutic Roles of Curcumin: Lessons Learned from Clinical Trials. AAPS J. 2013;15:195–218.

6. Aggarwal B.B., Kumar A., Bharti A.C. Anticancer potential of curcumin: Preclinical and clinical studies. Anticancer Res. 2003;23:363–398.

7. Lestari M.L., Indrayanto G. Curcumin. Profiles Drug Subst. Excip. Relat. Methodol. 2014;39:113–204.

8. Mahady G.B., Pendland S.L., Yun G., Lu Z.Z. Turmeric (Curcuma longa) and curcumin inhibit the growth of Helicobacter pylori, a group 1 carcinogen. Anticancer Res. 2002;22:4179–4181.

9. Reddy R.C., Vatsala P.G., Keshamouni V.G., Padmanaban G., Rangarajan P.N. Curcumin for malaria therapy. Biochem. Biophys. Res. Commun. 2005;326:472–474.

10. Vera-Ramirez L., Perez-Lopez P., Varela-Lopez A., Ramirez-Tortosa M., Battino M., Quiles J.L. Curcumin and liver disease. Biofactors. 2013;39:88–100.

11. Wright L.E., Frye J.B., Gorti B., Timmermann B.N., Funk J.L. Bioactivity of turmeric-derived curcuminoids and related metabolites in breast cancer. Curr. Pharm. Des. 2013;19:6218–6225.

12. Maria L.A.D.vLestari, Gunawan Indrayanto. Chapter Three – Curcumin. Profiles of Drug Substances, Excipients and Related Methodology. 2014;39: 113-204.

13. Anand P., Kunnumakkara A.B., Newman R.A., Aggarwal B.B. Bioavailability of curcumin: Problems and promises. Mol. Pharm. 2007;4:807–818. doi: 10.1021/mp700113r.

14. Han H.K. The effects of black pepper on the intestinal absorption and hepatic metabolism of drugs. Expert Opin. Drug Metab. Toxicol. 2011;7:721–729. doi: 10.1517/17425255.2011.570332.

15. Shoba G., Joy D., Joseph T., Majeed M., Rajendran R., Srinivas P.S. Influence of piperine on the pharmacokinetics of curcumin in animals and human volunteers. Planta Med. 1998;64:353–356. doi: 10.1055/s-2006-957450.

16. Lin Y.G., Kunnumakkara A.B., Nair A., Merritt W.M., Han L.Y., Armaiz-Pena G.N., Kamat A.A., Spannuth W.A., Gershenson D.M., Lutgendorf S.K., et al. Curcumin inhibits tumor growth and angiogenesis in ovarian carcinoma by targeting the nuclear factor-κB pathway. Clin. Cancer Res. 2007;13:3423–3430.

17. Marchiani A., Rozzo C., Fadda A., Delogu G., Ruzza P. Curcumin and curcumin-like molecules: From spice to drugs. Curr. Med. Chem. 2014;21:204–222.

18. Banach M., Serban C., Aronow W.S., Rysz J., Dragan S., Lerma E.V., Apetrii M., Covic A. Lipid, blood pressure and kidney update 2013. Int. Urol. Nephrol. 2014;46:947–961. doi: 10.1007/s11255-014-0657-6.

19. Menon V.P., Sudheer A.R. Antioxidant and anti-inflammatory properties of curcumin. Adv. Exp. Med. Biol. 2007;595:105–125.

20. Panahi Y., Alishiri G.H., Parvin S., Sahebkar A. Mitigation of systemic oxidative stress by curcuminoids in osteoarthritis: Results of a randomized controlled trial. J. Diet. Suppl. 2016;13:209–220.

21. Biswas S.K. Does the Interdependence between Oxidative Stress and Inflammation Explain the Antioxidant Paradox? Oxid. Med. Cell. Longev. 2016;2016:5698931.

22. C.D., Ruffin M.T., Normolle D., Heath D.D., Murray S.I., Bailey J.M., Boggs M.E., Crowell J., Rock C.L., Brenner D.E. Dose escalation of a curcuminoid formulation. BMC Complement. Altern. Med. 2006;6:10. doi: 10.1186/1472-6882-6-10.

23. Jurenka J.S. Anti-inflammatory properties of curcumin, a major constituent of Curcuma longa: A review of preclinical and clinical research. Altern. Med. Rev. J. Clin. Ther. 2009;14:141–153.

24. Recio M.C., Andujar I., Rios J.L. Anti-inflammatory agents from plants: Progress and potential. Curr. Med. Chem. 2012;19:2088–2103. doi: 10.2174/092986712800229069.

25. Daily J.W., Yang M., Park S. Efficacy of turmeric extracts and curcumin for alleviating the symptoms of ioint arthritis: A Systematic review and meta-snalysis of randomized clinical trials. J. Med. Food. 2016;19:717–729.

26. Ajay Goel, Ajaikumar B. Kunnumakkara, Bharat B.Aggarwal, Curcumin as "Curecumin": From kitchen to clinic. 2008;75(4):787-809.

27. Kocaadam B., Şanlier N. Curcumin, an active component of turmeric (Curcuma longa), and its effects on health. Crit. Rev. Food Sci. Nutr. 2017;57:2889–2895.

28. Sharma R.A., Euden S.A., Platton S.L., Cooke D.N., Shafayat A., Hewitt H.R., Marczylo T.H., Morgan B., Hemingway D., Plummer S.M. Phase I clinical trial of oral curcumin: Biomarkers of systemic activity and compliance. Clin. Cancer Res. 2004;10:6847–6854.

29. Mhillaj E, Tarozzi A, Pruccoli L, Cuomo V, Trabace L, Mancuso C. Curcumin and Heme Oxygenase: Neuroprotection and Beyond. Int J Mol Sci. 2019 May 16;20(10).

30. Dean J, Keshavan M Asian J Psychiatr. 2017 Jun; 27():101-111.

31. Andrade C. J. Clin Psychiatry. 2014 Oct; 75(10):e1110-2.

32. Lopresti AL, Maes M, Maker GL, Hood SD, Drummond PD. J Affect Disord. 2014; 167():368-75.

33. Zhang L, Luo J, Zhang M, Yao W, Ma X, Yu SY. Int J Neuropsychopharmacol. 2014 May; 17(5):793-806.

34. Cuiqin Fan, Qiqi Song, Peng Wang, Ye Li, Mu Yang, Shu Yan Yu. Neuroprotective Effects of Curcumin on IL-1β-Induced Neuronal Apoptosis and Depression-Like Behaviors Caused by Chronic Stress in Rats. Front Cell Neurosci. 2018; 12: 516.

35. Shao S1, Duan W2, Xu Q2, Li X3, Han L2, Li W2, Zhang D1, Wang Z2, Lei J2. Curcumin Suppresses Hepatic Stellate Cell-Induced Hepatocarcinoma Angiogenesis and Invasion through Downregulating CTGF. Oxid Med Cell Longev. 2019 Jan 16;2019:8148510.

36. Ikram M, Saeed K, Khan A, Muhammad T, Khan MS, Jo MG, Rehman SU, Kim MO. Natural Dietary Supplementation of Curcumin Protects Mice Brains against Ethanol-Induced Oxidative Stress-Mediated Neurodegeneration and Memory Impairment via Nrf2/TLR4/RAGE Signaling. Nutrients. 2019 May 15;11(5).

37. Park KS, Yoon SY, Park SH, Hwang JH. Anti-Migration and Anti-Invasion Effects of Curcumin via Suppression of Fascin Expression in Glioblastoma Cells. Brain Tumor Res Treat. 2019 Apr;7(1):16-24. doi: 10.14791/btrt.2019.7.e28.

38. Roxo DF, Arcaro CA, Gutierres VO, Costa MC, Oliveira JO, Lima TFO, Assis RP, Brunetti IL, Baviera AM. Curcumin combined with metformin decreases glycemia and dyslipidemia, and increases paraoxonase activity in diabetic rats. Diabetol Metab Syndr. 2019 Apr 30;11:33.

39. Tsvetkov P, Asher G, Reiss V, Shaul Y, Sachs L, Lotem J. Inhibition of NAD(P)H:quinone oxidoreductase 1 activity and induction of p53 degradation by the natural phenolic compound curcumin. Proc Natl Acad Sci U S A. 2005 Apr 12;102(15):5535-40.

www.ingramcontent.com/pod-product-compliance
Lightning Source LLC
Chambersburg PA
CBHW030738180526
45157CB00008BA/3232